The Group Fitness Survival Guide: 2019 Edition

THOMAS EMMETT

Look for this book and more on my author page at:
https://www.amazon.com/author/thomasemmett

CONTENTS

CHAPTER 1: INTRODUCTION TO GROUP FITNESS

My main purpose in writing this book, is to help and instruct those who are either considering teaching, or who are just getting started teaching. I also encourage those who have been teaching, even for many years, to pick this book up and read it, because you may find something that will help you to improve your classes. Keep in mind though, this is not a book about how to teach, as I only cover some basic information. It is mainly a reference guide to be used along with some type of instructor training class. The best way to learn to teach is by doing it, and actually practicing. Hopefully I can help you with that.

What group fitness is, what it is not

I will be the first to tell you, though teaching is often a high paying job, it is not, and can never be, a full time career. I doubt that even the healthiest person in the world can teach 40 hours worth of classes a week, for life. There might be someone out there that can do a single 40 hour week, but that cannot last forever. Teaching classes puts a lot of strain on the body and the voice. It will require more rest, and a higher caloric intake, if an instructor does teach a lot of classes each week.

This is a part time job, and the number of classes a person can teach is really determined by fitness level. If you are in better shape, you can teach more classes, or the other way around. I started off teaching 1-2 a week, and as my fitness level improved, I added more. In the last year I have spent most weeks teaching 8-12 classes, and it has really put a strain on me. But at the same time, I have never been in better shape. I would not recommend a lot of people teach this many classes. Start small, sub when needed, and try not to have a lot of regular weekly classes.

I mentioned fitness level, but the type of classes you can teach, will also determine how many you have. Most instructors start with one or two that they really want to do, and increase from there. Make those your specialty classes, and as you gain more experience and become more comfortable with teaching, learn to do others. Your starting classes should be the ones that you really want to do, and you should work hard at making them the best that you can. When I first started, step was my favorite, so I started with that one. Then, I expanded into strength classes, water aerobics, kickboxing, and finally cycle.

Instructors are made, not born

Everyone is not born to be an instructor. You might take classes for years before deciding to start teaching. You might know all the moves, be able to stay on beat, and have whole routines memorized, but once you put that microphone on and stand in front of a group for the first time, you will see it is not as easy as it looks. There is a lot to remember, a lot to think about, and you might just forget everything you had planned to do. It happens. But once you start planning your classes, practicing your breakdowns, and actually talking into the microphone in front of a group, it will get easier.

When I went through instructor training, I must have come up with about six step combinations in about ten minutes. I knew the moves, I could come up with a combination in a minute, but then when I actually put on the microphone and went to the front to teach, I had nothing. I had no idea how to actually teach it. So all my combinations meant nothing, because I could not do anything with them.

So maybe you think you are too shy to teach. Maybe you think you are not in shape to teach. Maybe you are afraid of standing in front of groups. 99% of all instructors that I know, including myself, started off as quiet and shy. None of us start off in top shape, and many were afraid of being in the front. That is normal. But as you teach more, you become more comfortable, you get louder, and you get into the shape that you need to be in. Or that you want to be in.

Sure, there are some people who are already loud. There may be some who are in excellent shape. There may be some that have no fear. There may even be some who can come up with a whole class in a matter of minutes. Don't let it get to you. You may have some characteristic that puts you above many others, but that alone will not make you a great instructor, nor will it make people come to your classes. It helps, but it is not everything.

We need more practice

If I were in charge, I would have these four words

painted in large letters on the wall in the group fitness room. But since I am not, I will insist on repeating it to everyone who wants to, or is already teaching.

There is nothing more important in group fitness than practice. You can be in shape, you can be loud, you can have excellent classes planned out, but if you do not practice, it will all be wasted. I believe that 10% of teaching is know how, and the other 90% is practice. I would never use anything in a class that I did not plan out, and practice beforehand. It may work in your head, but it may not work when actually doing it.

You need to spend time putting together combinations, and not only that, you need to practice breaking them down. You need to practice it with the music you are going to use, so you will know that you can stay on beat with the routine. You should practice talking as well. Talking while breaking down helps, because you not only learn the best way to break it down, but you also learn the best time to say what comes next.

I know we are busy, and there is not always time for practice. But think about this. You can write down your routines and look at them while teaching, but if you practice enough, you will not have to. Practice creates confidence, and it gets your routine into your head and body. You have enough to think about when teaching, but imagine not having to stop and think about what comes next during your class. Many times I have forgotten my combinations, gotten off beat, and came to parts where I had no idea how to break it down, all because I did not practice enough beforehand. I have also attempted combinations that I have used with a certain music speed with another music speed, only to find it did not work out. I simply refuse to do something now that I have not practiced, and know for sure will work out.

A word about winging it, or just making it up as you go. Unless you have been teaching for a long time, and know that you can put a class together while teaching, do not even think about trying this. This is especially true for cardio classes like hi lo, step, and even kickboxing. At this point, I am confident I could make up routines as I go, but I would rather not. If I do it for any class it would be kickboxing, but certainly not step or hi lo. It may not hurt that much to put a routine together while teaching, and using some moves that you find will not work, but the participants will likely know that you are making things up, and they may feel you are wasting their time. The time spent trying moves out, could have been spent on doing a routine that was already set.

Respect is earned

There are two things that I will talk a lot about. Practice and respect. Respect is indeed earned when teaching, and it comes largely from practice. Think about this. People take time out of their busy day, when they have a million other things to do, to come to *your* class for a workout. They come to *your* class rather than going to the gym, running on a track, swimming in a pool, or playing a game/sport, because they believe and trust that *you* can give them something better than they can get elsewhere. They do not have to come, but they want to.

Knowing this, it is *your* duty as an instructor to give them your best. This means putting on some good music, being excited to be there, and talking with your people. Having practiced your routine and knowing what you are there to do, you actually *do* the workout with them, rather than talking them through. Participants tend to think more of an instructor who participates with them. So do it, rather than just telling them what to do. They come to work, and many give you all that they have, so you ought to give them the same.

Sure, some people are not as in shape as others. You might have a class full of beginners, or you may have a very small class, maybe even two or three people. But no matter what, you help them get through it. You should teach with the same effort and intensity to two people, as if you are teaching to hundreds, and they will love you for it. That is how you get people coming back, by giving your all no matter what. I understand it can be disappointing to have a small class when you worked so hard on a new routine, but it happens, and they still deserve your best. That is how you earn respect.

Lead by example

I would be a bad instructor if I did not mention that by being an instructor, you will be put in a position of authority and popularity, and people will be watching you. You will find that many people will know who you are and what you do, even if you do not know them. As a health leader, people expect you to lead by example. This means getting in and staying in the best shape that you can be. If you hate exercise, you need to find something else to do with your life.

How can you expect to lead these people who are trying to get in shape and better themselves, if you yourself are not showing them the way? You ought to be in the gym, you ought to be exercising. Now, I understand that nobody is perfect, that life is hard, and that we all have problems. Maybe you are overweight. That's fine. The point is that you are trying to do something about it, instead of just sitting around eating junk. Nothing wrong with drinking a little if you feel the need, but you should not be going out and getting drunk in public, because a lot of people know you as an instructor, even if you do not know them. Maybe you have a problem with smoking. I know many who do. But if you are going through packs a day, people are not going to listen to a word you say. I mean, why should they quit smoking, while you continue to do it?

I had decided a long time ago that I would never have the people in my classes do something that I cannot do myself. How would it look if you have your class doing a certain exercise, and you are not doing it with them because you cannot? Either get in shape, or do something else until you are able to do it, and then bring that exercise back. Like I said, you have to earn it.

I am not talking about appearing to practice what you preach. Living right in front of others, and then in secret doing everything that you say people should not do. Get your heart and mind right, and your actions will follow. Then the people will follow you because of it.

Instructor interaction

I mentioned before that respect must be earned from participants, and other instructors. But that does not mean that you should disrespect your fellow instructors in any way. Whether you are new to teaching, or have been for a long time, there are just some things you should never do. You should get this in your head now, so it will not become a problem later on.

You will notice that when I am teaching instructor training, and give you the microphone to teach, I will do exactly as you do, whether it is right, or wrong. Many new instructors, even outside of training, will watch me in their class to see what I am doing. But know that anything you do, I am doing as well. So if you are off beat, I am off beat too.

I would never try to embarrass you in any way, because it is your class. If you are wrong in some way, I trust you will figure it out, and make it right. But I would never call you out, or go up to the front and do it right, so that others see that, and think less of you. I was once a beginner as well, and I know that it is only natural to make mistakes. This goes not only for new instructors, but for any instructor, as even I still make mistakes.

Should you find yourself in a class where the instructor is having a hard time, or makes some mistakes, talk about it afterwards in private. Feedback is always appreciated. If I am doing something wrong that I am not aware of, I would like to know. I might even need to know how to fix it, so get some suggestions ready.

Teaching is a hard job, and a difficult skill to perfect. So help your fellow instructors, rather than hurting them. If you are in a class that you just do not like, do not whine and complain, and talk about how bad the class is. Get through it, or leave if you need to, but be nice, and talk to the instructor about it after.

2019 Edit...

I did not change much in this chapter from 2009. Only made some minor fixes, but the content is still the same. Everything is still true, and I still agree with it today.

CHAPTER 2: BASIC CLASS FORMATS

This chapter is not exhaustive, but I do want to mention some of the essentials of your basic class types. If you can teach these four, you can teach anything, as most classes are a combination of the following. Certain classes such as yoga and pilates are exempt from this rule, but those such as cycle, athletic conditioning, cardio-sculpt interval, and water aerobics are not.

Most classes are about an hour long, though some express and strength classes are thirty minutes each. No matter what class you teach, they will all have a basic format. You start with a warm up, which should be light exercise designed to get your blood pumping and your muscles ready to go, followed by your workout, and then you finish with the cool down and stretching, which brings your heart rate back to normal. I notice some older instructors still tend to do some stretching at the end of the warm up as well, and you can do that if you want, just be sure you do the warm up first before stretching. I usually just do a longer stretch routine at the end, rather than two short ones, but it is the instructor's choice.

In general, it is best to do a warm up according to the class you are teaching. If you are doing step, run through some basic step moves. If the class is kickboxing, go through the basic punches and kicks. Hi lo works as a warm up for any class, but I find it more efficient to do the basic moves for the class you are teaching. That way, if there are new participants in your class, you will not have to stop and go through the basics during your class. Hopefully they will catch on in the beginning. For classes that are mainly strength, I would do a hi lo or step warm up, using basic moves only, just to get the blood moving. Usually for a strength class you would use a step anyway, so why not use it for your warm up too?

Hi lo impact

Most people nowadays probably have no idea what this is. I used to take a lot of these classes when I first started in early 2000, but I rarely see a whole hi lo class anymore. I really like hi lo, and one of my near future goals is to learn to teach one of these classes. If you do not already know, this is basically like a step class, except you are on the floor, and do not have the step.

This is a cardio class, and usually you would use faster music than you would in step, since there is no bench to trip over. Hi impact moves would be those such as jacks, where both feet leave the floor at once, and lo impact moves would be those such as marching, walking, and step touches, where there is always at least one foot on the floor. Hi lo is just a combination of all of those moves.

Some basic hi lo moves include: March, walk, step touch, grapevine, jog, knees, ham curls, jacks, shuffles, and lunges. The good thing about hi lo is that you are not limited with staying on a step. Any of these moves can be done in any direction, and you can have the class move throughout the whole room if you wanted.

If you wanted to spice up your hi lo routine, feel free to add in some step moves. Sure there is no step in front of you, but you can still use V steps, turn steps, and travel knees, along with many others. If you can make it work, you can do it. You might even feel the need to add some kickboxing moves. Perhaps make it a hi lo and kickboxing type class. It is your class, do what you will.

Step

I believe step is the very first class I ever took. I know it was the first I ever taught. I liked step since the beginning, and for some reason which I do not know, step has always been easy for me to follow. I find that many people have a hard time in step classes these days, and I can understand why, because I am starting to struggle as well. The problem is not so much the step, but the classes have become a lot more complicated.

When I started with step, the music was slower, the moves were easier, and the instructors only used a few combinations in a class. Nowadays, the music speed is increasing, the number of combinations in a class is increasing, and in some cases the risers are getting higher. A number of step classes I have taken in the last few years seem to be more dance than step. I have gone to some classes, and even I had no idea what was going on.

I teach step in the old style, using slower music, easier moves, less combinations, and I spend more time breaking them down. Step can be hard by itself, and many people struggle with it. I do not like to lose people in my class, so I try to help them see it is not that hard. Once you learn the moves and how the instructor breaks it down, as all are different, step is easy to do. Remember this when you are teaching it.

This is also the one class you do not want to have people coming in late to, because they will miss some combinations, and that will mess them up for the rest of the class. So, encourage people to come on time. Also, I strongly suggest you do basic step moves for a warm up, rather than hi lo.

Some basic step moves include: Basic step, V step, turn step, over the top, A step, L step, across the top, straddle, and various travel moves, which can be knees, ham curls, kicks, etc. Travel moves could also be in various repeater numbers, such as 3 or 7. Step is like hi lo, and you can add such hi lo moves as jacks, lunges, step touches, and grapevines to your routine.

Step is also like hi lo in combination design, and breakdown. I will talk more about this in Chapter 4, but a combination in Hi lo or Step will be 32 counts. Or 32 steps if you prefer. You will start your combination with the right foot leading, and when finished, you should end with the left foot ready to start the same combination again.

As far as breakdown goes, many instructors seem to do the next move, or few moves repeatedly, until it is learned, and then do the same for the next move, before putting them together. I find it easier for everyone if I do one move at a time, alternating with a basic step in between, and once they have it, doing the same thing with the next move. Then I'll put them together and go from there, repeating the process. It is basically what works for you. Everyone has a method that works, and that is what you should use. That of course, will be found with practice.

As far as making your classes interesting, sometimes the traditional horizontal single step will not cut it. Sometimes you will need to turn it vertically. Sometimes you may want to add a second bench in, maybe have three or four benches. You can really arrange them anyway you want to, so long as you make it work. Just remember, those benches run out quickly as you use more steps, so do not plan a multi-step routine unless you are certain that everyone can get what they need.

I should mention a couple of safety issues with step. It goes without saying, but make sure that all risers are hooked in correctly so nobody trips. Make sure shoes are tied, make sure the whole foot comes up on the bench, and make sure there are no loose objects nearby, or on the floor, that can get in the way. I have had a few people trip in step. I have even done it myself. So, encourage them to watch their step as well as you, and to raise or lower risers accordingly. Faster music means lower benches, and slower music allows for higher if you choose. Just be sure to mention that they can adjust their risers, if they need to. I would not use more than 3 risers on each side, and only for slow music if you do.

Kickboxing

For some reason, kickboxing has always been my hardest class to teach over the years. I could put together some combinations fairly easily, but when I actually tried to teach them, I could not get it right. I just kept getting off beat. But after teaching a lot of kickboxing classes for almost a year, I finally got it. Since then, kickboxing has become my best, my favorite, and my hardest class to take.

Kickboxing is a lot simpler than step, and for many who struggle with step, I encourage them to take this class, as there are only a few moves that you need to know. It is just a matter of putting them together differently. As far as music goes, step should be the slowest, hi lo should be the fastest, and kickboxing should be in between. I will mention specific speeds, and talk more about music, in the next chapter.

Kickboxing can be taught in different ways. It could be taught like a hi lo or step class, with a long, continuous routine. Or, it can be taught as I currently do, using just 8 count combinations at a time. I tried for so long to teach it like a hi lo class, and it failed miserably. But doing 8 count combinations at a time works perfectly for me. You could also mix some hi lo in when appropriate, but you certainly would not mix step with this class.

Basic kickboxing punches would include your jab, cross, hook, and uppercut. Basic kicks would be your front, side, roundhouse, and back kicks, along with knees. Some instructors would also add in crescent kicks as well. You can also add in various elbows, blocks, hand strikes, and head butts, along with ducks and jumps. It helps a lot to have a martial arts background as I do, but it is not necessary. It just gives you more to work with, so long as you can make it work in a class.

The only way I can think of to make your class harder, is to make it like a boot camp class. You can add in various stations, either all cardio, or some cardio and some strength, like pushups and crunches. It is really up to you what you want to do, as there is a lot of variety in the way instructors teach kickboxing. You should consider how many people are there, and how much equipment you have. Generally, kickboxing classes are larger, so it is not always convenient to get equipment out, and have people moving around in stations. You can always add in place stations like I do, such as jacks, lunges, football runs, and jumps. That way you are not short on equipment, or space.

Strength/toning

Out of the four class types here, this is certainly the easiest class to teach. There is no complex choreography unless you want there to be, so you are free to do anything really. You can go with the music, or you can do timed exercises or stations, letting people work at their own pace. Certain exercises you will find work better one way or the other, so you can always do a combination of the two. This is where you are likely to find 30 minute classes, such as abs or lower body, which tend to be quite popular. The hour classes tend to be for the whole body, and you should work it all. I would stay away from doing any, or a lot of cardio. Except for the warm up, unless this is an athletic conditioning, or boot camp type class. And if the class is only 30 minutes, no extra cardio should be done.

In these type classes, you get to take out a variety of equipment. This of course depends on what you have to work with. Even if you have a lot of equipment, these classes can get large, and you can run out. You can give people options if needed, like using dumbbells or a barbell to make it work. In these classes you can use various barbells, dumbbells, exercise bands, medicine balls, Physio-balls, mats, gliders, core boards, steps, and anything else your gym might have.

There are 8 main muscle groups that you should work, according to your class type. The 4 large muscle groups should take first priority, and those would be the legs, back, chest, and abdominals. The 4 small muscle groups should take second priority, and that would be the calves, shoulders, biceps, and triceps. The smaller muscles will be worked by working the larger ones, so if you are short on time, work the larger ones.

If you wanted to break the groups down some more, say if you have a lower body class, you can do that, and work each part. For the legs, you have the quadriceps in front of the thigh, the hamstrings behind the thigh, the inner and outer thighs, the gluteus, and the calves. Not trying to get into the names of all the muscles, as there are many, but you could also break up the back into upper, middle, and lower. The shoulders can be divided into the front, side, and back. There are exercises that work all parts of a muscle, and there are exercises that work a certain part of a muscle. At least try to do the ones that work the whole muscle at once.

If you choose to do this class with the music, you can do single reps again and again, or you can mix things up. For every exercise you can adjust how fast or how slow you work, according to your music. Of course for these classes you would be using slower music, a little more so, or the same as you would for step. You can do single lifts, all the way up and down, or you can do: 2 counts up, 2 down; 3 counts up, 1 down; 1 count up, 3 down; 4 up, 4 down; half way up and down; half way down and up; or you can hold certain moves in the middle, or even do tiny pulse lifts. You learn which exercises work best with what count combinations by practice, of course.

There are a lot of safety concerns with this class, and I cannot possibly list them all here. Basically, you need to keep an eye on your class, and mention safety cues as you teach. You teach enough, and you will say them naturally. Always watch, and check people for correct position. In this class type, I give you permission to walk around, and check people. You do not always have to be in the front, doing every exercise with everyone. With step and hi lo, you better be doing it with them, because they cannot do it without you. But for strength, you are free to move. Sometimes you may just have to get next to someone, and do the exercise until they get it right.

Also, make sure everyone is doing the full range of motion. Not partial movements, or swinging the weights around. If you see swinging, have them grab something lighter. Proper form is better than heavy weight any day of the week. Make sure the guys understand that, because the class is not weight lifting like it is in the gym, and they will attempt to lift heavy on you, only to find out they cannot do it. Do encourage proper breathing as it is quite necessary, and mention body alignment cues as needed.

It helps if you are also a personal trainer, or have experience weight lifting, because you will certainly know more exercises to use in a class, than those who do not lift weights. But it is not necessary. Having taken an Anatomy and Physiology class will also help a lot. Make sure that when teaching these classes, you try and use common names for muscles and groups, rather than using their actual names, whether you know them or not. I tried to avoid using actual names here because of this. You can talk about the quadriceps, or the latissimus dorsi when teaching, and have people look at you funny, or you can just simply say you are going to work the legs and back.

2019 Edit...

I have actually been teaching full hi lo classes for many years now. At the time of the original book I was only hoping to do so, but now it is no problem for me at all. Kickboxing, though hard to figure out at first, is quite easy now as well.

I only discussed the four main class types here. By now, there are so many more that exist. Even back then, I could have done a section on cycle, and one on water aerobics. But I tried to focus on the main ones that you have to know in order to teach anything else. You could easily take the ideas you have learned by now, and make them work in a cycle or water aerobics class.

CHAPTER 3: MUSIC IS EVERYTHING

I mentioned a lot in previous chapters about planning out your classes and practicing them beforehand. But there is something else that is needed, and that is good music. After all, if you did not have music, you would not have a class.

You will find that many people often compliment you on your music rather, than your class. Instructors tend to use certain types of music in their classes, and you will usually have participants who see this, and come to your class because of it. As far as importance goes, music ranks up there with practice and planning. It is necessary that you keep it new and keep it hot, if you want to have a smooth class.

Keep in mind before reading this chapter, that I will give you several recommended speed ranges. These numbers vary slightly from what you will hear when getting certified. They are not wrong. There are just no real set speeds, which is why you are given ranges. Follow my principles as I give them, and you will be fine.

Music speed according to classes

If you could only have the minimum number of CDs to get by with when teaching, you would want something in 130 bpm and 140 bpm. Beats per minute is something you would need to look at when shopping for new music, as each class requires a certain number. As I said, you can teach any type of class you want if you only had something in 130 and 140. Naturally, a higher number would mean the music is faster, and a lower number would mean it is slower.

In general, when you are starting to teach, you would want to use something slower, because it will help you as you think, and try to remember what comes next. It also helps you with your breakdown, so you are able to stay on beat and cue what is next. Then when you get more comfortable, you can increase the speed if you choose. Faster music will often result in more sweat, and more calories being burned as you are moving faster. But just as there are minimum speeds to be effective, there are maximum speeds as well.

The slower music classes would be step, and any strength based classes. For strength classes, I would recommend working in the 126-132 bpm area. Especially if you are working with the music, rather than doing timed exercises. Step you can work a little faster, with speeds ranging from 126-136. I think 130 is best, but I have recently increased to 136, because I feel my step classes can go there, and I am comfortable with the speed. With step though, there is an inverse relationship between music speed, and bench height. Slower music allows for higher steps if you choose, but with faster music you need to reduce the height, because it will be impossible to keep up and stay on beat. There is a greater chance of tripping with fast music. I would also make the moves easier too.

I have heard of some step classes these days that go faster than 136. I have heard of 140, and even 150, and I have no idea how someone would do that. I think it is unsafe to do so. I suppose that at that speed you would have to use the bench alone, with no risers. I certainly would not recommend anyone to go that high, especially beginners, but if you have been teaching for a while and can safely make it work, I will not stop you from going there. If you can stay on beat and do it safely, and the participants can follow you, then have at it.

The faster music classes would be kickboxing, and hi lo. For kickboxing, I would suggest starting at around 135 bpm, and then you can go up as you please. As kickboxing is a more difficult class to teach, it is easier to start slow and move up, as you are comfortable. My kickboxing range for you would be 135-144 bpm. I started at 135, and slowly worked my way up to 138,140, and at the moment, 144. I have no intentions of going any higher, as my current set up works best with this speed.

There are some instructors who would go above 144 in kickboxing. Some may do 150, and I have even taken some classes that do 160-170. As with step, increasing the speed would generally mean easier, and more basic moves being used. You cannot do the same combinations at 144, as you can with 160. I found out that I have combinations I used to do at 135, that do not work at 144. As I said, if you can make it work, stay safe, stay on beat, and the people can follow you, do what you are comfortable with.

The last class I will talk about is hi lo. This one has the greatest range of speed, but it is very much like kickboxing. Since you are on the floor and there is no equipment around, you are free to go high on this one. The same principle applies though. Start slow until you are comfortable, and increase from there. Your conditioning should really determine what you could do here. My suggested range would be 135-160. I would use 144 like in kickboxing, but that is really because I have a lot of good music at that speed. I can be comfortable going to 150. Finding music above 150 is hard to do, but it is out there, if you so choose.

I want to leave you with some final words about music speed. I gave you a range for each class type, and you are free to go outside of that range, but keep a few things in mind. If you choose to go slower, your participants will likely not be challenged, and may end up leaving your class. It has happened to me. If you choose to go faster, it might become unsafe, and they might not be able to keep up with you. This will also result in them leaving. I know some people who will not go to a certain class because it is too fast.

If you do stay within the range, start at the lower end until you are comfortable, and move up as you choose. You will notice that you will have to make some changes as you change your speeds. Certain moves or combinations do not work at every speed. Your breakdown may also have to change if your speed does. The key here is to practice your routine with the music, so you are certain it will work.

Shopping for music

Let me be the first to tell you that buying music will be expensive. But it is necessary. You can expect to spend $15-$25 per CD. You cannot just take any old CD and put it on for class. It does not work that way. You need to get special music that is mixed, is continuous, and that has a smooth, consistent, and noticeable beat. There are several sites online that sell music for group fitness, and I will mention some of those shortly.

That leads to something very important that you need to be aware of. Never buy a CD, and then just pop it in for a class without ever listening to it first. When you buy something new, make sure you listen to the whole CD at least once, preferably a few times, before you use it. Also, make sure that you actually practice with that CD as well. You may find during this time that the CD is not very good. It may be filled with songs that after listening to them, you really do not like that well.

The main reason to listen before you use, is that certain CDs can throw you off beat if you are not careful. Sometimes you will find songs that seem slower than the rest, and are played at half speed. This tends to happen with faster music. With some slower music, there may be songs that are played faster, or double time. The beat is still there, and the music is still at the same bpm, however you can be thrown off by it. There are other times still when the song becomes silent for a few counts. I have a CD that does that, and if you are not ready for it, the whole class may stop completely on you, or get off beat. And sometimes, you might just have one of those songs in there that nobody knows or likes, and it just needs to be skipped over.

Music websites

There are four main websites online where I buy music from, and I want to briefly discuss each one. There are other sites out there, but most sell the same CDs, so there is no point in mentioning them, but you are free to shop around. These sites are current at the time of my writing this, and may change in the future. And no, I am not getting anything out of mentioning them, I am just answering the question that you are bound to ask, and that is, "Where can I buy my music from?"

Many sites have a few things in common. You can usually shop online, order a paper catalog, and listen to samples before you buy. You can order CDs from them, and now many sites are having downloadable versions made available for a few dollars less. New music tends to come out every few months at least, or with some places having new music added weekly. You can also create your own custom mixes if you are willing to pay. Here are the sites.

www.powermusic.com
www.dynamixmusic.com

I am grouping these together because they are very similar in what they offer. You can buy online, or get a catalog to mail in an order. You can see the music, and listen to samples online. Downloads are also becoming available for both sites for a little less. These sites offer the largest variety in music types and speeds, and the CDs tend to be excellent. You would almost have to try to get off beat in a class. The beat is consistent and clear, and beginners should shop here.

The problem with these sites as I see it, is that the CDs are set, and you cannot choose your speed. You basically have a CD with whatever speed it comes in, and you cannot change that. New music also comes out a little slower here than other sites, with new CDs coming out every few months or so. If you hear a brand new song on the radio, you likely will not get it here for several months.

www.cardiomixes.com

I actually shop here the least, but it is not because they do not have any good music. Their music is usually a little cheaper than the first two sites, and I do not believe downloads are available right now. You can listen online before you buy, and for some CDs you can choose your speed, but most are set. This site comes out with new music about as often as the others, and they have a good variety to choose from. They also do not sell out, or have to backorder CDs, unlike the first two, when new music comes out. You cannot get a catalog from this one either.

instructormusic.com

This site is perhaps my most frequented as of late. I get a lot of my kickboxing music here, because this is the only place where you can choose your speeds, and 144 bpm is not found anywhere else. Here is where you will likely find brand new songs before any other. New CDs come out each week, and you can also download here. The way this site works is that with each song set that comes out, you can choose your speed, and there are several choices. Say a new CD comes out. You can choose to get that CD in 128, 130, 136, 144, or 150 bpm. I like this because if you have a good CD in one speed, you can get it in another speed for another class, if you choose.

What makes this site good is also what makes it bad, I think. As there are multiple speed choices for each CD, you will often find many songs at either half speed or double time, and that is why you need to listen before you use. The beat is not always 100% clear and easy to find either, and you may get off beat in a class.

I recommend this site for more advanced instructors, and the first ones for beginners, but you are still free to check out any of them, as there are good CDs available at all of the sites. All sites have their advantages and disadvantages, but if you know what you want and what you are looking for, you will be able to find it.

Last words about music

Because music is so important to teaching, I want to conclude this chapter by mentioning yet again a few things you need to remember. Stay within my recommended speed ranges. Go slower if you need to, go faster if you are able and choose to, but keep it safe. Always practice your planned routine with your planned music, and make sure to listen to it before using it.

Music is expensive, so feel free to share with other instructors. Do make it a point to use your own music the most, because that is what makes your classes, and sets them apart from the rest. Always used mixed music rather than regular songs with breaks in between, so that everyone can stay on beat, and so that the class will run smoothly.

Think about your location as well, and remember that though it is your class, it is not really about you, it is about the people. You have certain types of people at different gyms that like different types of music. If you are at a gym, and the people clearly like pop/hip hip, do not put a rock CD in. If they want dance/techno music, do not play a country CD. Consider your audience, because they will not stay, and may not come back, if you play something you should not. So buy a variety of music types according to where you are teaching, and they will love your class.

2019 Edit...

Music has changed a lot in 10 years. Back in those days, we had just gotten rid of cassette tapes. CDs were the main source of music, and MP3 players were starting to be used. iPods were new, but most people used CDs.

These days, CDs are rare, though I still use them. Now it is mostly phones, iPads, or laptops that people tend to use. I have over 200 CDs at this point, and I have no plans to change to anything else.

My music speeds are also different now. I pretty much use either 136 bpm or 144 bpm for everything. It has been like this for a long time now. For cycle, step, water aerobics, and strength classes, I use 136 bpm. For kickboxing, hi lo, and boot camp classes, I use 144 bpm. I never could have used these speeds when I first started teaching, but by now I have been doing this for about 16 years.

The music websites have changed some too. The big thing now is making your own music. I only really buy from Power Music now. Each of the sites still sell CDs like they always have, but now they have mixing programs that you can use to make your own. You choose the songs you like, choose their speeds, choose their order, and even choose the number of songs in a mix. Then you pay for what you make, and download it. I put those mixes on CDs after that.

With Power Music, you pay for each song, and then you own those songs, so you can reuse those in other mixes if you want. The limit here is that most of their songs come from already existing CDs that they sell. As time goes, they seem to come with other versions that you can also use. I have so many CDs at this point, that I really do not buy or make much anymore.

I did check all four of the websites in this chapter to be sure they are all currently working. The last website

has gone through some address changes, so I found
and added the most current one on here for you.

CHAPTER 4: COUNTING, CUEING, STAYING ON BEAT

Counting and cueing is something that you will cover a lot when training or getting certified for group fitness, and I will not go into great detail with it here. You really need to have an instructor with you, actual music playing, and you need to be practicing in person. I do not expect that by reading this you will fully understand the proper way to count and cue, though if you have been taught already, it should help. I am including this section because it is an important part of teaching, but I do not expect you to fully understand it unless you are already teaching.

You know that you need continuous mixed music in

order to teach. This music is created at a certain beat per minute. It allows you to have an organized class, and to teach at the same rate throughout, rather than just moving at any speed, which could get ugly. If you have taken classes regularly for any length of time, you will soon find yourself being able to find and stay on beat with the music, sometimes even when the instructor loses it. You may not always know exactly what is going on, but you just know you are doing it right.

Combination basics

Combinations in step, hi lo, and perhaps kickboxing, are made up of 32 counts each. Usually, as in step or hi lo, there will be 32 steps, or movements of your legs, to equal these 32 counts. A full 32 count worth of moves would give you one combination. You would normally start the combination with your right leg moving first, and you will end it so that your left leg will start the left side of that 32 count combination. So, to do the whole right and left side will give you 64 counts total, and then you are ready to move to the next. Each side of your combination will be the same, just the leading leg will change on your moves. It is basically looking at where you want to go, and then coming up with a move that will get you there, in however many counts you have to work with.

For step and hi lo, your combinations are generally made up of 4 and 8 count moves. You would start on the right leg, and do any combination of moves you want, so that you will end up ready to repeat them with the left leg starting next. So, you could have a simple combination made up of four 8 count moves, or you can make it more complicated by adding in several 4 count moves. Keep in mind, it is harder to do a lot of 4 count moves rather than 8, and it is also harder to cue a lot of 4 count moves, as you may wind up talking continuously the whole time. If you can do it however, then have at it.

Sometimes, you may find it easier to group several small moves together into a large 16 count combination, and create a name for it. I have a few of these I use in step, and it is easier to teach as one, than to name each move separately. I mainly did this because breaking them down further would have caused me to end somewhere I did not want to end, or it would have caused me to get off beat. Then I would have to get off beat several times when breaking it down. So, sometimes you need to be creative to save yourself some trouble.

Kickboxing can be different than step and hi lo, depending on how you want to make it. I mentioned before that making 8 count combinations work best for me. I will do one combination on the right side, and then repeat on the left, before doing a new one on the right again. If you can do it, go ahead and put a 32 count combination together, and teach it the same as you would for step or hi lo. I tried to do this, but it will not work for me. It may for you.

Kickboxing is a little different though, as you have different hand and leg movements, rather than 4 or 8 count moves like in step. Any hand movement, any type of punch, elbow, or block, is normally 1 count per move. Kicks, and possibly knees, are usually 2 counts apiece.

So if you wanted to do an 8 count combination, you could use 4 punches, followed by 2 kicks. That will give you the 8 counts. These are minimum however. If you want to take more time with a punch or kick you can do so. You can make a punch last for 2 counts and a kick for 4, depending on what you are trying to do. If you want to allow for some rest, or maybe you are adding in a duck or a jump, or something that will require some time to get back into position, you can do that.

Putting your combination to music

If you are new to teaching, the first thing you should listen for is a beat. If you have trouble finding it, you can try turning the bass up. You can also compare speeds by playing something around 128 bpm, which will be fairly slow, and then something at 140 or faster right after, and you will notice the difference between them. You should also test out your combination while listening to your chosen CD, to see if you can both find and stay on beat. This beat should be consistent throughout the CD, and that is where you want to be.

I have music from many years ago, where the beat was very clear and easy to find. For some reason, the beat is not so easy to find anymore. But do not worry. Though the beat may be hard to find at times, the music will always be phrased in 32 counts. It used to be easy to hear that as well, as there always used to be a cymbal type of sound at the start of each 32 count phrase. The music also tends to work up towards the end of the 32 count, and then it starts off the next.

Your combinations should start when the music begins a 32 count, but it is not absolutely necessary. Since you will be breaking down your combinations, you will still be on beat, but you will likely deviate some from starting on a 32 count. That is fine, so long as you try and get back there again, when doing the whole combination from the beginning. It helps you and the participants to stay together, because they will also recognize the 32 counts in the music, as well as the beat, so they can follow you easier.

Counting down and cueing moves

When you teach and break down your combinations, you always want to count down from 8. Start with 8, and work your way down to 1. You can also start at 4, 16, or 32 if you so choose, as those are just different multiples of 8, and will keep you on beat. I use the higher numbers occasionally when doing jacks or knees, mainly to make it seem like you are doing a lot, but you could really just count down from 8 a few times instead.

You should never say 1 when counting down, but rather you should say what move is next. Sometimes, if you have a lot to say, or the music is faster, you may want to leave out 2 or 3 as well. Do not forget to still do those moves, even though you are telling them what is next.

You will eventually find yourself talking according to the beat of the music, and will give sufficient notice of what comes next. As I said before, you ought to practice counting down and cueing with your routine, as you will find the best way to do it before you get in class.

When I first started teaching, I would count everything. I had to, or else I would lose track of what I was doing. Say, if I was doing basic steps. I would do 8 on the right and then 8 left, and then drop it down to 4 on each side. I would always count out loud every step I did. I did this to make sure that I stayed on beat, did not lose count, and so that I knew I was doing an even amount of moves on each side. I also did that so that everyone would stay with me, and do as I did.

Eventually, as you become comfortable, you do not have to count every move you do. It takes a lot more energy and breath to count everything in a class. Once you become familiar with your music and can easily find the beat, you can just listen to the music and know how many counts you have left, so you will not actually have to talk all the time.

Right now I still count a lot, but not as much as I used to. My purpose now, is so I know I am doing an even amount of exercises on each side. It just would not be right to do 32 knees on one side, and 24 or so on the other, for example. I also like to do it to keep people on beat, and together. Counting helps a lot when you do not want to lose anyone, and that is also why I do it, because it makes the class easier to follow.

CHAPTER 5: HOW TO GET PEOPLE IN, AND KEEP THEM COMING

I want to start off by saying that this is one major part of teaching that you do not have complete control over. You can have hot new music, you could have the best routines and hardest classes, you could always be on beat and never make a mistake, and yet you can still have small classes. Accept it now, that no matter how much work you put into teaching, you cannot make people come to your classes. Getting people to exercise is a hard task for anyone. You cannot use class size as a measure of how good you are as an instructor, though usually the better instructors will have larger classes. There are several factors that will determine your class size, and I want to list as many as I can think of, as there are many indeed.

Class demographics

First, you have to consider the class type. Some classes are more popular just because of what they are. From what I have seen, the most popular classes seem to be super abs, cardio strip, kickboxing, and funky fit. This of course is also dependent on certain factors, such as gym location. Certain classes do better at certain gyms, based on what population you have. Funky fit may be the favorite at one gym, while kickboxing may be at another.

You also have to look at the day and time. People tend to take classes on certain days and at certain times. Typically, classes are more popular later in the day, around 5:00-7:00 pm. This seems to be common at all gyms. Popular days can vary, but I would say that the middle of the week tends to work the best, meaning Tuesday, Wednesday, and Thursday. This is not definite however, as people still go on other days.

Looking at your actual class makeup, you will see that the majority of participants are women. Men tend to lift weights in the gym, while the women take the classes. When you do have men in a class, it will usually be in kickboxing, cycle, or super abs. Participant ages also vary, and do so by gym and class type. In one location you could have a lot of older participants in a yoga class, for example. But in another location, yoga might be made up of younger people. There really is no set rule for who will take what class.

I almost forgot to mention, but the time of year also affects group fitness. You have holidays, exam weeks, vacations and breaks, and even bad weather or traffic can affect class size. Even if you are the best instructor in existence, there will be times when you may even have nobody show up, but this is completely normal, and nothing to worry about. People have lives and other things to do besides taking classes, which are not absolutely necessary to life, so you would do well to remember that.

Lastly, class size can also be determined by the amount of equipment available. There is usually a set amount of bikes or weights, or anything else you may try to use. If you only have twenty bikes, you cannot be upset if there are not thirty people in your class. You can get creative at times, perhaps by having people use either a barbell or dumbbells, but you will still be limited somehow. You may even have to tell some people to either take another class, or try to get there earlier next time. But you will learn which classes fill up the fastest, and be able to let people know appropriately.

It is not everything, but it is important

A large determiner of your class size is indeed based on the instructor, as the instructor really makes the class what it is. Let us say you have a popular class at a perfect time, and on the right day. People will come to your class for a few reasons.

You are first of all excited to be there. You try to get to know your people, and you talk to them when possible. People can tell when you are glad to be there, and they do not want to hear you saying you do not want to be there, or else they might not stick around. You also interact with people during class, encourage questions and comments, and persuade them to come back and bring friends. You also laugh and make jokes, and have a good time. This would be your personality that they want to see.

They also want to see your preparation. People do not want to see an instructor come in, and have nothing planned out for the day. They certainly do not like stopping during the class while you figure out what you want to do next. They also do not like you stopping and playing with the music, changing CDs constantly and such, as they are here to work, not rest. That is why you should be using continuous mixed music, so you will not have to do that. This is why you practice your routine while playing music and by talking, before you come to class. If you prepare properly, you will not forget your combinations, and make a fool of yourself in class. So practice, practice, practice.

So you have personality, and you are prepared to teach. But what about your actual plan? Do you have an appropriate warm up, workout, and cool down, according to your class and population? Every gym and every class is different, so you may have to change your routine to fit the class. Perhaps in one gym your class may be too hard, while in another, that same routine may be too easy.

You need to be able to make changes according to what you are working with. This is a hard skill to have. But we must all work towards being able to have a plan, and being willing and able to change it when things go bad. Sometimes you just might have to throw a combination out the window if they just cannot get it right.

Preventing discouragement

As you have seen, there are many factors that determine your class size. What really matters is that you give all that you have with what you have to work with. You ought to teach a class of four people just the same as you would with a class of sixty. Now, you might be disappointed when only four people show up after you worked so hard coming up with a new routine, but you cannot overlook them and see it as a wasted effort. You have to earn your people, and it may be that those four like your class so much that any time they see your name in the future they are there, no matter what class it is. Then they might start bringing friends and telling others about you, and your classes will grow. You never know what could happen.

It is hard starting off as a new instructor, or even in a new gym, even though you are not new to teaching. It takes time for people to learn your style and get to know you, and eventually they will. You should also take sub opportunities as they come, as that will allow you to show other people and other classes what you are about. You might wind up getting some of those people into your classes if they like you. Remember what I said, respect is earned around here.

This can be a hard issue for some who just start teaching, and expect that they will have the largest class out of them all. Do not be disappointed if that is not the case, as it may take years of teaching before you have the biggest class. You may even teach your whole life, and still not have a large class, but that should not be the measure of how you good are as an instructor.

Spreading the word

You can help get more people in your classes, or just simply into any class, by talking about it outside of the gym. If you know people who go to your gym, tell them about the classes. I am a personal trainer as well, and I make it a point to tell all of my clients about the classes, because they are usually free with a gym membership. Unlike personal training, which is extra. Classes are basically free, group personal training. And even though you do not think a person can survive one of your classes, that should not stop you from telling them about others.

There is a class made for everyone. People just have to find what works for them. Encourage people to try different classes according to their abilities, and what their goals are. You have your cardio classes, meant to burn fat and calories, such as kickboxing, step, cycle, and athletic conditioning. You have your strength classes, designed to build and/or tone muscle, such as Group Power, super abs, HABIT, and booty/belly.

You have your flexibility/toning classes, like yoga and pilates. You also have your fun classes, which can also be considered cardio, like funky fit, Zumba, hip hop, and cardio strip. Encourage them to try different ones, and see what they like.

2019 Edit...

The most popular class for a long time now has been Zumba. No matter what gym I go to, Zumba has always been the winner when there are multiple choices at once. It is the one most likely added, and kept on a schedule. It is most likely to be done each day of the week. And it is probably going to have the highest numbers, and the most regular attendees.

CHAPTER 6: PREVENTING BURNOUT, AND GETTING CREATIVE

I cannot possibly overlook burnout, as it can become a serious issue with teaching. If you have taught for any length of time you have probably experienced it, and hopefully you have overcome it. Or maybe you are there now, and are looking for a way out. It happens to everyone at some point, and it has happened to me several times. I want to take this word apart so that you will know how it happens, and how you can overcome it. As I have.

What burnout is, what it is not

Burnout is simply when you just get tired of teaching, and you do not get excited about doing it anymore. I suppose there could be different degrees of burnout, though I have not experienced them all. It is mainly a mental problem, though I can see how getting injured could make it a physical one as well. Like if you are teaching more than you can handle, and you get hurt.

As a mental issue, you get tired of teaching, and it affects your classes negatively. You do not put much effort into creating a routine. You likely do not practice it as much as you should beforehand, and you start making mistakes in class.

People see that you do not really want to be there, and likely you will fail to motivate them. They may not want to be there either. You feel like you are doing the same thing all the time, and you cannot come up with anything new. You are just plain bored with your classes. But how does it come to this? I think there are several reasons for it.

How burnout occurs

I know for a fact that I cannot teach the same class at the same gym, more than once a week, without getting burnout after a while. It may be possible if you do it on two separate days, with two separate times, with two completely different groups of people. But that is still risky. Too much of the same class can also lead to injury.

The problem is when you teach the same two classes at the same gym. Say, kickboxing on a Monday and Wednesday at 5:30. The thing that really gets the burnout started, is when you have the exact same group of people that come to both classes. I cannot even imagine doing that more than twice a week.

After a few weeks, maybe a few months of doing this, you are guaranteed to get burnout. You find yourself doing the same routines all the time, and you have a hard time coming up with anything new that you have not done already. You use the same music, and you come to think that your same group of participants are bored as well. You lose that motivation to teach, and that is how it happens.

Over the years, this has happened to me on two separate occasions. One with step, and one with kickboxing. So I guess you can say I have gotten burnout two times. But I have overcome it each time. If you want to overcome it as well, there are a few things that you need to realize, and some changes that you need to make.

Conquering burnout

First of all, do not put yourself in a position to get burnout. Do not teach the same class more than once at a single gym. You can sub when needed, but leave it at that. If you teach at multiple gyms, feel free to teach the same class at each one if you choose. You ought to have a whole different group, which may result in a whole different class. Be careful here though, because you may have three or four gyms you teach at, and even with a single kickboxing at each gym each week, that is four classes a week, and will get you burned out rather quickly. Though the people will not get tired of your routine, you probably will.

This leads to something I mentioned before, but need to mention again. Burnout is mainly a mental problem. Even if you teach the same class multiple times each week at the same gym, with the same people, just because you get tired of it, does not always mean that they are too. The fact that the same people are coming each week, may mean that they are not tired of it, but chances are they will be eventually if you do not change your routine. You can always ask for thoughts and suggestions, and see what happens. But even if they are not bored with the same routine, it is better practice to give them different ones so that they can avoid the plateau, which will likely occur from doing the same exercises.

Now, let us say you do have burnout, and the people are bored with your classes. There are several ways you can go about this. You can give up a class, or choose to alternate weeks with someone else, so that the people can get a break from your routine. Or you can choose to take some time off from that class, and let someone else take them for a while. What you choose to do may either help you or your participants, or it may help you both.

Another technique you may try, is to start taking classes yourself. You can see how other instructors teach, and it may encourage you to change how you teach as well. You might also learn some new moves or combinations that you can play with and use in your class. It is best if you have access to other gyms to take their classes. You are less likely to find people that take your class there, so any moves you learn will be new at your gym.

If you are teaching a class like step, there is yet more that you can do to improve your class. You can always add another bench, and do double, triple, or even quad step. Just be aware of class size, and equipment amount. Adding more benches or changing their arrangement, allows you to create new moves that you cannot do with just one bench. There is really no reason to get burnout in step, because even if you still use the same old moves, you can change orientations and bench amounts, so that it is slightly different.

Speaking of changing classes, you ought to change your music, and buy new music when you are able. You may also decide to change your speed, as that will make a class different. You might even be able to combine class types a little more. Perhaps use more hi lo moves in your step class, or take some step moves and use them in hi lo.

If you combine your class types, there is no limit to what you can do. I have even done different types of stations in kickboxing, which actually made it more like an athletic conditioning class, but it works, and they like the variety. It may be that people cannot get to athletic conditioning, and would like to do some in kickboxing.

It is up to you to conquer burnout, and you should do it by any means necessary, short of quitting teaching completely. You can change your class, your music, or just plain take a break from that class, if that is what you need to do. But if you are determined to overcome, then you will, and you can get back to teaching that class again one day.

You should also be aware of seasonal changes. At certain times of the year, the people that come to different classes will change, for whatever reasons. So you will not have the same group around forever. Even if you just need to survive until a semester is over, do what it takes to get there in one piece.

The thought just came to me, and I do not know why I never thought of it before, but if you are having a hard time, just talk to your other instructors about it. We have all been there, and we can help each other through somehow. You may be surprised to find that another instructor has tons of material you can use, even if he or she is not actually teaching the class in question, and you can learn something new. Just do not give up, no matter what.

CHAPTER 7: TIPS, TRICKS, TEACHING TECHNIQUES, AND AVOIDING MURPHY

If you have somehow managed to get through life without meeting Murphy, I can assure you that you will meet him when teaching, perhaps many times. I am referring of course to Murphy's Law, which says that anything can and will go wrong. You can be a veteran instructor, have the best music and classes, and have large amounts of regulars who follow you to every class you teach, but something can still go wrong. The idea is that you want to practice and prepare as much as possible, but that includes much more than I have mentioned already in previous chapters.

Preparing for anything

First of all, make sure that you have sufficient travel time. You are likely to find an accident, or some type of event on the road that you did not expect, that would cause you to be late to class. This also means that you should not fill up your schedule with more than you can handle. Ideally, you should be able to get to your class early enough to get prepared, and be ready to go on time. It is likely that the one day you are running late, is the day there will be an accident or construction or something else.

It has to be said, but also make sure and use the bathroom before going to class. You are going to have a hard time getting through an hour class when you have to go to the bathroom 20 minutes in.

Speaking of preparation, you are almost always provided with a microphone and stereo systems. But sometimes, something does not want to work. Always bring two extra sets of new batteries for the microphone you will be using, because the day you do not have any batteries with you, is the day the ones that are there will be dead. You certainly do not want to teach a step class without a microphone. I assure you of that. But still, even if you have your batteries, there are times when the microphone does not work, and you do not know why. This is rare, and should be reported immediately to someone who can fix it. Sometimes though, you just have to turn the music down, and get it done without.

Speaking of music, remember what I said about listening to your music first? You also want to make sure your CD works where you intend to use it. I have two new CDs I just downloaded that work everywhere except for one gym, and I cannot figure out why, because the CD player is exactly the same. So, test your music in the location you intend to use it, before class time.

Always carry backup music with you, so you are not stuck with nothing. But then, there may be a time when the CD player is broken, and will not play anything. Same with the microphone, do what you can do until it is fixed. You ought to check everything, along with all switches if the player is not working. I have found that some switches were in the wrong place before, and that made all the difference.

If you need a microphone belt where you teach, I would also recommend buying and bringing your own. Even if there are a lot to use, you may need it one day, if you do not choose to use it all the time. Along with that, if you sub a lot, or even if you teach a lot, you should keep an extra change of clothes or two in your car. This will prevent you from needing a trip home for more workout clothes, if you need to teach another class that you did not plan on doing. And if you do use your emergency clothes, do not forget to replace them when you get home. The same goes for your batteries.

Speaking of preparation, you ought to bring some water with you to class, and drink whenever possible. Some classes require a towel like cycle, or a gel seat, but it depends on the class and how much you sweat. Do bring some Gatorade if you are teaching multiple classes in a day, as this will prevent cramps. I find I can survive two hours worth of classes without cramping, but it will happen on that third hour without some Gatorade. You will learn what you can handle, but I would suggest starting that Gatorade early if you know you will be teaching for a while. There is nothing worse than having your quadriceps cramp during jacks, halfway through kickboxing. So plan ahead.

Along with that, make sure you do eat something before class, so you have something to work off of. It should not be a lot, unless you eat a while before class. Just make sure you can handle and digest the amount. Being hungry with 45 minutes left of class is not pleasant. And do eat something after as well. I would avoid soda or anything with caffeine before class, as that will dehydrate you more, and you do not need any more of that. But let us say you had that soda. Did you remember your Gatorade?

Small changes to help you survive your classes

Though I have said before that you ought to be in top shape if you want to stay an instructor, you do not have to be when starting out, and it is not expected of you. You get there by teaching more, and exercising on your own. In the event that you are not able to survive your own class, there are ways that you can make it easier to get through.

You should start teaching a few classes a week, perhaps no more than three. That will depend on your ability, if you are in shape or not, and how much those classes are needed. Eventually you can do more if you choose, but I will say that it is not easy, no matter how good a shape you are in, when you start doing more than six or so. I can say that because I have done 8-12 classes a week for most of the last year, with most of them being hour classes, and it is not much easier than when I started. But you do notice the difference in your ability when that number drops.

If you are teaching strength classes, it is a little easier to get by than in heavy cardio classes, like step and kickboxing, though there are shortcuts to all of them. I do not recommend you always do what I am about to say, as you will only be cheating yourself, but it is up to you. These techniques are really for those who are out of shape, and really have a hard time getting through a class, along with those who teach too much. Here you go, but do try and keep this information confidential from your participants, as these are instructor's secrets.

With strength classes, this one is obvious. You do not have to use the maximum amount of weight you can handle. You can use lighter weights, easier bands, and if you give options, you can take the easier route. You could also walk around more, rather than staying in the front, and doing every exercise with the class. These classes you can usually do this, unlike in step, where you have to do the whole class with them, because you are basically just doing a single movement multiple times, and they will not get lost.

You could also create various timed stations, or just do timed exercises, letting them go at their own pace. This frees you up to walk around, and make sure they are doing it right, rather than causing you to do it yourself, though you should still do some when possible. This works for any class. I actually taught super abs like this for the first year I think, by rotating through stations. My reasoning was because the class was large, and I wanted to do something different than everyone else, but it was also partly because I did not think I was ready to do a whole thirty minutes of abs myself. I shortly got rid of that setup, because I felt I wasted too much time demonstrating each station when the exercises changed, but it is still a good beginner setup.

With step and other classes, you can adjust the difficulty, but it takes some more thought to do. For step, you can always lower your risers until you stop getting out of breath. Remember that increasing bench height makes the class harder. Much more than increasing music speed. Which brings me to the other technique.

You can always change the music speed. For any class, if you use slower music it will be easier than using faster music. Many gyms have tempo control now, so you can still use the same CD, and either speed it up or slow it down, as you need. Of course you cannot use the tempo control for a large speed change, as it will not sound right, so just use another CD if you need a big change.

I want to finish this section by saying that the previous techniques are temporary solutions to a problem. You should not use light weights or slow music forever. You are supposed to be leading by example, and how would you like explaining to your class why you are using three pound weights, while they are all using eight or more?

Your last option, and desperate measure that you can take, is to talk them through the class while doing nothing at all. This should be avoided at all costs, unless you have no choice. The only reason you should ever do this is if you are very sick, and could not get a sub. But if you mention that in the beginning, they may voluntarily cancel the class for you, and let you go home. There will be no excuse for not being prepared, or having any clothes, because you know by now that you should have had an extra set of clothes in the car.

I will grant you permission to not teach, if for some reason you are teaching for most of a day. I think I have taught up to four, hour long classes in a single day. I would say that if you do more than 3 hours in that short of time, you should be able to take it easy, but it still depends on the type of class. It's really up to you, and what you are able to do.

Tips for improving your classes

I cannot stress it enough, that you need to take other instructor's classes when are you able. It is here that you learn how other people break down their combinations, if you are having trouble breaking them down yourself. It is here that you can learn new moves that you can use in your classes. There is no stealing amongst instructors, only borrowing. Sometimes, you might see something you like, so you can take that, play around with it, modify it if necessary, and use it in your own class. Perhaps you might take a little from several classes and add it to your own, putting it in with your own material. Feel free to take what you think is best, and use it. After all, there are only so many different punches and kicks you can do, and so many combinations of them.

I would suggest taking sub opportunities as they are asked of you. This is especially important for new instructors, because you will become more experienced in those classes, and perhaps be able to teach them regularly yourself in the future. Subbing also allows you to meet participants who likely do not know you or take your classes already, whether you are new or not, and if they like you, you may have some new faces in your classes. So subbing is an opportunity for improvement, getting more people into your classes, and sometimes, it may lead to you teaching more, or teaching different types of classes in the future.

As far as actual teaching goes, do not worry about other instructors so much, and how they teach. You may find that more experienced instructors move around the room a lot, they will mirror occasionally, or all the time, and they never seem to make a mistake. Get it in your head that you are supposed to mess up at times. It happens. Sometimes a lot. But that is why practice is so important, to minimize those mistakes.

It does not matter how long a person has been teaching, you can still mess something up. I have been teaching a long time, and I do make mistakes occasionally. The key is to pick yourself up, get back on beat, and keep the class moving, because most of the time nobody will even notice.

There are times when it may be hard to come up with enough material for a class. It might be that you are new to teaching, or perhaps you are starting up a new class that you have not taught before. It takes creativity and practice to come up with enough to fill a whole hour, since you are limited in the number of exercises you know, and you are not sure how much you can do in that time. Suppose you are starting off with a kickboxing class, but you do not have an hour worth of material. With most new instructors, I suggest putting together a routine with as much as you can come up with, and then add some abdominal work at the end, or any other muscle you want. Most people tend to finish off with abs, but you could really do anything, even something different each week, if you choose.

To show you how it would work, here is a sample class. Let us say you start with a 5 minute warm up, and finish with a 5 minute cool down. Say you have 35 minutes of kickboxing material. That leaves you with 15 minutes to do anything else you want. You might even do half abs and half legs. It is your class. You can do what you want with it. And eventually when you learn more, you can add more kickboxing material in, and get rid of the toning part, or you can keep it the same. This technique also works well with step, and would with hi lo as well.

Concerning mirroring, I would suggest you avoid that until later. In the beginning, face the front, do what you are comfortable with, and stay there. Mirroring is facing the class, and doing the same move they are, but on the opposite side. This is best left for the advanced instructors, because you must remember to be on the opposite side of what you are telling them to do. So when they are doing a right jab, you will be saying right jab, but doing a left.

Certain classes you do not want to mirror in however, and step is a major one. They need to see where you are and what you are doing, or you will lose them. Step is hard enough for most people to follow. I would also say that hi lo should not be mirrored, but it is a little safer to do than in step. If you practice with it.

I think that the only real limit to teaching well is how comfortable you are with it. You become more comfortable by practicing, by being prepared, and by teaching a lot. Most instructors start off quiet and shy, but as you become comfortable, that will change. Group fitness actually will improve your public speaking abilities, and you will find that it is easier to be in front of other groups as well.

Though you should not mirror right away, you should use the mirrors that are in the room to help you teach. You and your class ought to be facing them, and that way you can keep an eye on them. It helps because you do not have keep looking behind you to see what it going on. Using the mirrors is very important when teaching, because you can see when they are with you, and when they are not. It also helps if you are nervous, because you do not have to look directly at everyone.

The next step

So maybe you have been teaching for a while now, and are looking for something new. You took my advice and picked an easy class to start with, like super abs, and you worked towards teaching the class you originally wanted to do, let us say step. Now you can teach that one perfectly as well. You want something more. Well, here are your options.

By now you have probably subbed for various classes, and have some ideas of what you might like to teach. You could keep the cardio and choreography route, and expand into hi lo or kickboxing. You could go the strength route, and start teaching some type of strength class. You could do something completely different, and do some yoga or pilates, or perhaps cycle or water aerobics. You might even want to get into a dance class of some type. If you teach long enough, you will eventually move into other classes, usually whether you want to or not.

As I said before, I started with step, and then quickly went right into super abs, water aerobics, and HABIT. I think water aerobics was the only one out the three that I actually did want to get into, and I had never even taken a HABIT class before that time, so I just did what I thought should have been done. Kickboxing was added next, and I did want to teach that one, along with cycle. I was not too excited about cycle, but as with the rest, once I worked with it and came up with some good material, I liked it. I can happily teach any of these classes now, and am looking to expand into something new.

Hi lo has been my goal since the beginning, but those classes are so rare nowadays, that I have a hard time putting a routine together, because I cannot see how others do it. But I am determined, and hopefully one day I will be able to do it. I would also like to teach hip hop, but that one will be my greatest challenge, and will remain my long term goal. With hip hop, I can break down the moves and teach it, and I can find some hot music, but I am limited because I cannot make up any moves. Nor do I know what to call them. I can take a class, and both learn and do a routine well after a lot of practice, but that is it.

So think about what you have done, and what you would like to do, and make it a point to go there. Just as everyone has a certain class that they are best at, you will see what you cannot do well just the same. So even if you are limited to a few classes, strive to make them the best that there is, and people will know you as the kickboxing instructor, or the cardio strip instructor, or whatever it may be.

You do not have to teach every class in existence, and I hardly know anyone who does. Take what you have to work with, and bring it. Remember these words, and repeat after me. "We need more practice."

ABOUT THE AUTHOR

Thomas Edward Emmett Jr lives in a small town in NC. He currently works as a nurse, and as a group fitness instructor. He has been writing for most of his life, but this is his first published book. Besides work, he is finishing up his fifth degree. In his free time he enjoys writing, playing video games, fixing his house, and spending time in the mountains.